SELF HEALING WITH BIOFIELD TUNING FORKS:

An Introduction to Using Tuning Forks

By Shani Riviere
Copyright © 2023 Shani Riviere LLC
All Rights Reserved

TABLE OF CONTENTS

Introduction to Biofield Tuning - pg. 6
Brief History of Biofield Tuning - pg. 8
Understanding Sound Healing - pg. 10
The Science Behind Vibrational Sound Healing - pg. 12
Tuning Fork Therapy - pg. 15
Types of Tuning Forks - pg. 16
Weighted Tuning Forks vs Unweighted Tuning Forks pg. 20
Benefits of Using Different Types of Tuning Forks - pg. 22
How to Use Tuning Forks for Self Healing - pg. 24
How to Use Weighted Tuning Forks - pg. 27
How to Use Unweighted Tuning Forks - pg. 28
Your Tuning Fork Session - pg. 31
Tuner Frequency Table - pg. 32
Techniques - pg. 34
Harmonic Frequency Tuning Forks pg. 38
Planetary Frequency Tuning Forks pg. 41
Choosing the Right Fork - pg 45
Using Tuning Forks for Specific Ailments - pg. 47
How To Use Tuning Forks For Stress and Anxiety - pg. 49
Using Tuning Forks for Sleep Disorders - pg. 50
Using Tuning Forks for Digestive Issues - pg. 52
How to Use Tuning Forks for Meditation & Mindfulness - pg 54
How to Use Tuning Forks for Chakra Balancing - pg. 56
How to Use Tuning Forks for Energy Healing - pg. 57
Precautions to Take While Using Tuning Forks - pg. 59
How to Maintain and Care for Your Tuning Forks - pg. 63
Final Thoughts - pg. 65
A Letter to you - pg. 66

Chapter 1: Introduction to Biofield Tuning

Ah, bio-tuning forks! The perfect tool for those who want to tune their bodies like a musician tunes their instrument. But don't worry, you won't have to practice scales or arpeggios with these bad boys. Bio-tuning forks are actually a set of specially designed forks that are calibrated to emit specific frequencies that can help restore balance and harmony to the body.

Think of it like as a symphony for your cells - each fork representing a different instrument in the orchestra, playing its own unique note to create a beautiful, harmonious melody. And just like a conductor, you can use the bio-tuning forks to guide your body back into perfect pitch. So if you're feeling a bit out of tune, don't fret - just grab a set of bio-tuning forks and get ready to harmonize your way to wellness!

Chapter 2: Brief History of Biofield Tuning

The history of frequency vibration and biofield tuning is a fascinating journey through the evolution of sound and energy healing practices.

The use of sound and vibration for healing purposes dates back thousands of years to ancient civilizations such as the Egyptians and Greeks, who used sound in their religious and healing ceremonies. In the 20th century, scientists like Nikola Tesla and Albert Einstein explored the relationship between frequency and energy, laying the foundation for modern theories on quantum physics.

The Solfeggio frequencies, which we will touch on later, are a set of six tones that were used in ancient Gregorian chants for healing and spiritual purposes. History has it that the tones were lost for centuries until a group of mystical healers rediscovered them in the 1970s and began using them in their healing practices.

In the 1990s, a woman named Eileen McKusick began studying the body's biofield, a subtle energy field that surrounds and permeates the human body. She discovered that by using tuning forks calibrated to specific frequencies, she could help release blockages and tension in the biofield, leading to improved physical and emotional well-being.

Since then, biofield tuning has gained popularity in the alternative health community, with practitioners using tuning forks to help balance the body's energy field and promote healing. While the scientific evidence for biofield tuning is still evolving, many people have reported positive results from this unique and non-invasive form of energy healing. Who knows where the future of biofield tuning will take us, but one thing's for sure - it's a fascinating and ever-evolving field.

So, whether you're a skeptic or a believer, there's no denying the power of sound and vibration to influence our bodies and minds.

Chapter 3: Understanding Sound Healing

Tuning forks have been used for centuries as a healing tool, and there are many benefits to incorporating them into a wellness routine.

First and foremost, tuning forks work by creating a vibration that can be felt in the body. This vibration helps to release tension and blockages in the body's energy field, promoting deep relaxation and stress reduction. It's like a gentle massage for your energy field!

Sound healing is the practice of using different sound frequencies to promote relaxation and improve physical and emotional well-being. It may sound like a bunch of woo-woo, but trust me, it's more than just an excuse to bang on a gong or play with singing bowls.

The idea behind sound healing is that every part of our body vibrates at a certain frequency, and when we're sick or stressed, our vibrations get out of whack. By using sound, we can help restore balance and promote healing.

Now, if you're thinking this all sounds a little too new-agey for your taste, don't worry. Sound healing can be as simple as listening to calming music or taking a few deep breaths. Or, if you're feeling adventurous, you can try attending a sound bath, where you lie down and let the soothing sounds of gongs, singing bowls, and other instruments wash over you. It's like a spa day for your ears!

Of course, not everyone is convinced of the healing power of sound. Some people might think it's all a load of hot air. But hey, if it makes you feel better, why not give it a try? Worst case scenario, you get to take a nap in a room full of cool instruments. And really, isn't that the dream

Chapter 4: The Science Behind Vibrational Sound Healing

Vibrational sound healing is a holistic healing practice that uses sound vibrations to promote physical, emotional, and spiritual well-being. The theory behind vibrational sound healing is that everything in the universe, including our bodies, is made up of energy and vibrates at a particular frequency.

When our body is out of balance, it can be due to blockages or disruptions in our energy flow, which can lead to physical or emotional imbalances. Vibrational sound healing uses sound waves to help remove these blockages and restore balance to the body's energy system.

The use of sound can affect the body in many ways, including through the vibration of cells and tissues. When sound waves enter the body, they can stimulate cells and tissues to vibrate at their optimal frequencies, promoting healing and restoring balance.

What's more, sound waves can also affect the brain and nervous system. The vibrations from sound can help reduce stress and promote relaxation, which can help boost the body's natural healing processes.

Studies have shown that vibrational sound therapy can be effective in reducing stress, anxiety, and pain, and improving sleep quality. It has also been found to have a positive impact on the immune system, helping to boost immune function.

In addition to promoting relaxation, tuning forks are also said to help improve circulation, boost the immune system, and support overall physical and emotional well-being. By restoring balance to the body's energy field, tuning forks can help alleviate a wide range of symptoms, from physical pain to emotional trauma.

Another benefit of tuning forks is that they are a non-invasive and non-pharmaceutical healing option. Unlike medication or surgery, tuning forks don't come with any unpleasant side effects or recovery time. They're easy to use and can be done in the comfort of your own home.

Vibrational sound healing with tuning forks is a practice that uses specially designed metal forks that vibrate at specific frequencies to promote healing and balance in the body.

When a tuning fork is stricken, it creates a pure tone that resonates at a specific frequency. When the tuning fork is placed on or near the body, the vibration from the fork is transmitted to the body's tissues and cells, stimulating them to vibrate at their optimal frequencies.

The vibrations from the tuning fork can help remove blockages in the body's energy flow, promoting healing and restoring balance to the body's energy system. The specific frequencies used in tuning fork therapy are believed to have different effects on the body and can be chosen based on the specific needs of the individual.

For example, the frequency of 528 Hz is often used in tuning fork therapy as it is believed to have a calming effect on the body and can help reduce stress and anxiety. This frequency is also known as the transformation and Miracles frequency as well as DNA Repair. The frequency of 432 Hz (also known as the OM frequency) is also commonly used and is believed to have a grounding and balancing effect on the body.

Chapter 5: Tuning Fork Therapy

Tuning fork therapy can be performed on specific points on the body, such as acupressure points or chakras, or can be used to create a field of sound around the body. The practitioner may also use multiple tuning forks at different frequencies to create a harmonious and balanced sound.

Vibrational sound healing with tuning forks works by using the specific frequencies of tuning forks to stimulate the body's tissues and cells to vibrate at their optimal frequencies, promoting healing and restoring balance to the body's energy system. The practice can be tailored to the specific needs of the individual and can be used to target specific points on the body or create a field of sound around the body.

While the scientific evidence for tuning forks is still evolving, many people have reported positive results from this unique form of energy healing. Whether you're looking to alleviate stress, boost your immune system, or simply relax and unwind, tuning forks may be just what the doctor ordered.

In summary, vibrational sound healing works by using sound waves to promote balance and harmony within the body's energy system. It has been shown to have a positive impact on physical, emotional, and spiritual well-being by promoting relaxation, reducing stress and anxiety, and improving sleep and immune function.

Chapter 6: Types of Tuning Forks

There are several different types of tuning forks used in vibrational sound healing, each with its own unique frequency and healing properties. Here are some of the most common types of tuning forks:

1. Solfeggio tuning forks: Solfeggio tuning forks are based on an ancient musical scale that is said to have powerful healing properties. There are six main Solfeggio frequencies, each of which corresponds to a different note on the scale. These tuning forks are often used to promote physical, emotional, and spiritual healing. The six Solfeggio frequencies include:

   UT – 396 Hz used to remove fear and guilt
   RE – 417 Hz used to undo situations and facilitating change/manifestation
   MI – 528 Hz as we mentioned before is used for DNA repair, transformations and miracles
   FA – 639 Hz used for connecting and attracting abundance and love
   SOL – 741 Hz used to remove toxins and negativity is also used for expression and solutions

LA – 852 Hz used for awakening intuition (852 Hz +963) Hz is the pineal gland activator

2. Chakra tuning forks: Chakra tuning forks are designed to correspond to the different energy centers, or chakras, in the body. Each chakra is associated with a specific frequency, and using chakra tuning forks can help balance and align the energy flow in the body.

3. Brainwave tuning forks: Brainwave tuning forks are designed to correspond to different brainwave frequencies, such as alpha, beta, theta, and delta. These tuning forks can help promote relaxation, reduce anxiety, and improve focus and concentration.

4. Acutonics tuning forks: Acutonics tuning forks are based on the principles of Traditional Chinese Medicine and are designed to stimulate specific acupuncture points on the body. These tuning forks can help promote healing and balance in the body's energy system.

5. Fibonacci tuning forks: Fibonacci tuning forks are based on the Fibonacci sequence, a mathematical pattern found in nature. These tuning forks are believed to have a harmonizing effect on the body and can help promote balance and relaxation.

6. Harmonic Tuning Forks: Harmonic Tuning Forks are based on the principles of musical harmony, using mathematically precise intervals such as the perfect fifth, perfect fourth, and octave. These intervals create harmonic relationships between frequencies known to bring the biofield into a state of natural resonance and coherance.

7. Planetary Tuning Forks: Planetary tuning forks are tuned to frequencies derived from the orbital and rotational cycles of celestial bodies, such as the Earth, Sun, Moon, and planets in the solar system. These frequencies are based on the concept of "cosmic resonance" and were popularized by Swiss mathematician Hans Cousto, who converted astronomical data (like the length of a planet's orbit) into audible sound frequencies.

Each type of tuning fork has its own unique healing properties and can be used in different ways to promote healing and balance in the body. Tuning forks can be used alone or in combination with other vibrational sound healing techniques to create a customized healing experience for each individual.

Chapter 7: Weighted Tuning Forks vs Unweighted Tuning Forks

Let me give you the lowdown on weighted vs. unweighted tuning forks. Weighted tuning forks are like the heavyweights of the tuning fork world. They have a little extra oomph and are designed to be held against the body for a longer period of time. Think of them as the bulldozers of the vibrational sound healing world. They are great for breaking through blockages and getting things moving again. One of the most popular weighted tuning forks is the OM which vibrates at a frequency of 136.10 Hz. It stimulates the heart chakra and is frequently used in meditation and healing.

On the other hand, unweighted tuning forks are like the featherweights of the tuning fork world. They are lighter and designed to be struck against a hard surface, such as a rubber block, to produce a pure tone. These tuning forks are more like the precision tools of the vibrational sound healing world. They are used off the body, either side of the head close to the ears or in the sound energy field of the area you are working on. They are great for targeting specific points on the body and promoting focused healing.

So, if you're looking to plow through some deep-seated blockages, go for the weighted tuning fork. But if you're looking for a more delicate touch to target specific areas, go for the unweighted tuning fork. Just remember, both have their own unique benefits and can be used in different ways to create a customized healing experience for each individual.

Chapter 8: Benefits of Using Different Types of Tuning Forks

There are many benefits to using different types of tuning forks in vibrational sound healing. Here are some of the key benefits:

1. Targeted healing: Different types of tuning forks can be used to target specific areas of the body, such as acupuncture points or chakras. This can help promote focused healing and balance in specific areas of the body.

2. Customized healing: Because different types of tuning forks have different frequencies and healing properties, they can be used to create a customized healing experience for each individual. This allows the practitioner to tailor the treatment to the specific needs of the individual.

3. Relaxation and stress reduction: Tuning forks are believed to have a calming effect on the body and can help reduce stress and promote relaxation. This can help improve overall health and well-being.

4. Improved energy flow: Tuning forks are believed to help promote the flow of energy in the body, which can help promote healing and balance.

5. Improved focus and concentration: Brainwave tuning forks are designed to correspond to different brainwave frequencies and can be used to promote improved focus and concentration.

6. Spiritual healing: Solfeggio tuning forks are based on an ancient musical scale that is said to have powerful healing properties, including spiritual healing.

Overall, the benefits of using different types of tuning forks in vibrational sound healing are many and varied. By using different types of tuning forks, you can create a holistic healing experience that addresses the physical, emotional, and spiritual needs of the individual.

Chapter 9: How to Use Tuning Forks For Self Healing

Now for the part you have been waiting for...How do we use tuning forks for self healing?

There are a few different techniques that you can use when using tuning forks for self-healing. Here are some of the most popular techniques:

1. Direct application: This involves holding the tuning fork directly on or near the body. For example, you might hold the tuning fork on an acupressure point or chakra to promote energy flow and balance.

2. Sound bath: This involves striking multiple tuning forks at once and allowing the sound to resonate throughout the body. This can be a powerful way to promote relaxation and balance.

3. Chakra balancing: This involves using tuning forks that correspond to each of the seven chakras to promote balance and healing in each area. You can hold the tuning fork near each chakra and focus on the corresponding sound to promote energy flow and balance.

4. Brainwave entrainment: This involves using tuning forks that correspond to different brainwave frequencies to promote relaxation, focus, or other desired states of mind. You can hold the tuning fork near the head and focus on the corresponding sound to promote the desired state

5. Interval training: This involves using two different tuning forks together to create an interval that promotes balance and harmony. For example, you might use a C and G tuning fork together to create a perfect fifth interval, which is believed to promote balance and harmony.

Chapter 10: How to Use Weighted Tuning Forks

Step 1

You will want to produce a sound in the weighted tuning fork by either using a rubber mallet to strike it or you can gently tap it on your leg or palm to create the vibration. (you will aim at the weighted portion of the tuning fork.)

Step 2

Do not strike the tuning fork on a hard surface as this may cause damage and/or break your tuning fork.

Step 3

Always hold your tuning fork by the stem but keep your wrists flexible.

Step 4

Use the tuning fork directly on the area of your body experiencing pain or that has any issues. Touch the area gently to allow the vibration of the fork to penetrate the area.

Chapter 11: How to Use Unweighted Tuning Forks

Step 1

You will produce a sound by using a rubber mallet or puck. If using a mallet, you will strike the fork gently at the top. If using a puck, you will strike your fork gently on the puck.

Step 2

Hold the stem of your fork with your wrists, arms and fingers relaxed.

Step 3

You will hold the fork at a reasonable distance from the ear then cross it over your head to the other ear to tune yourself to its vibration and then hold it over the area where you need healing.

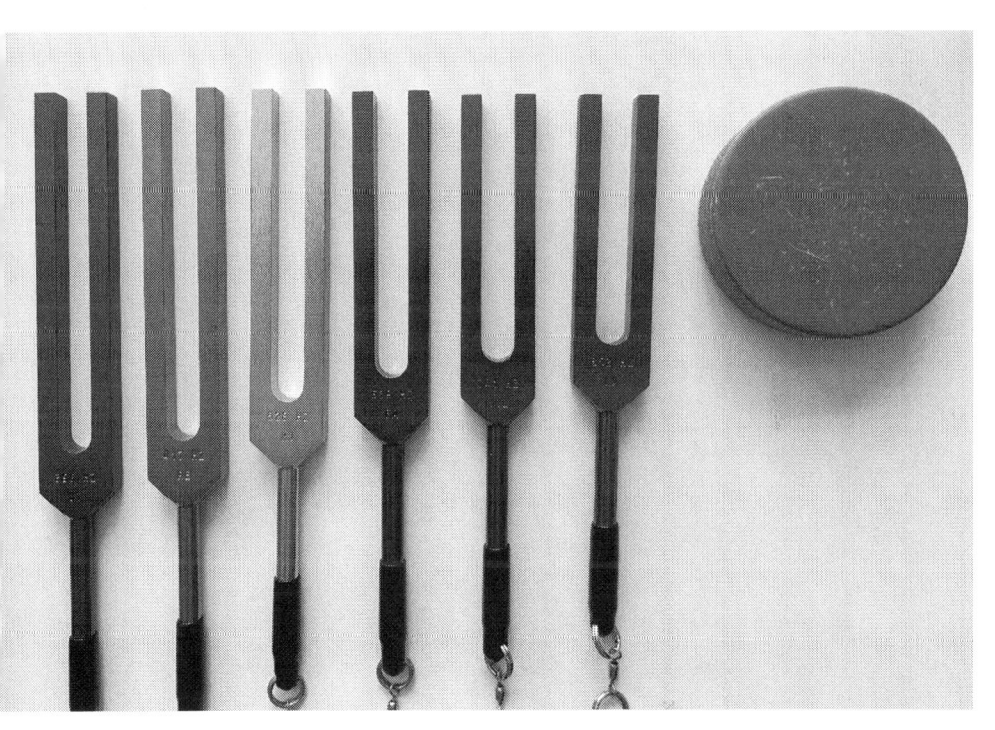

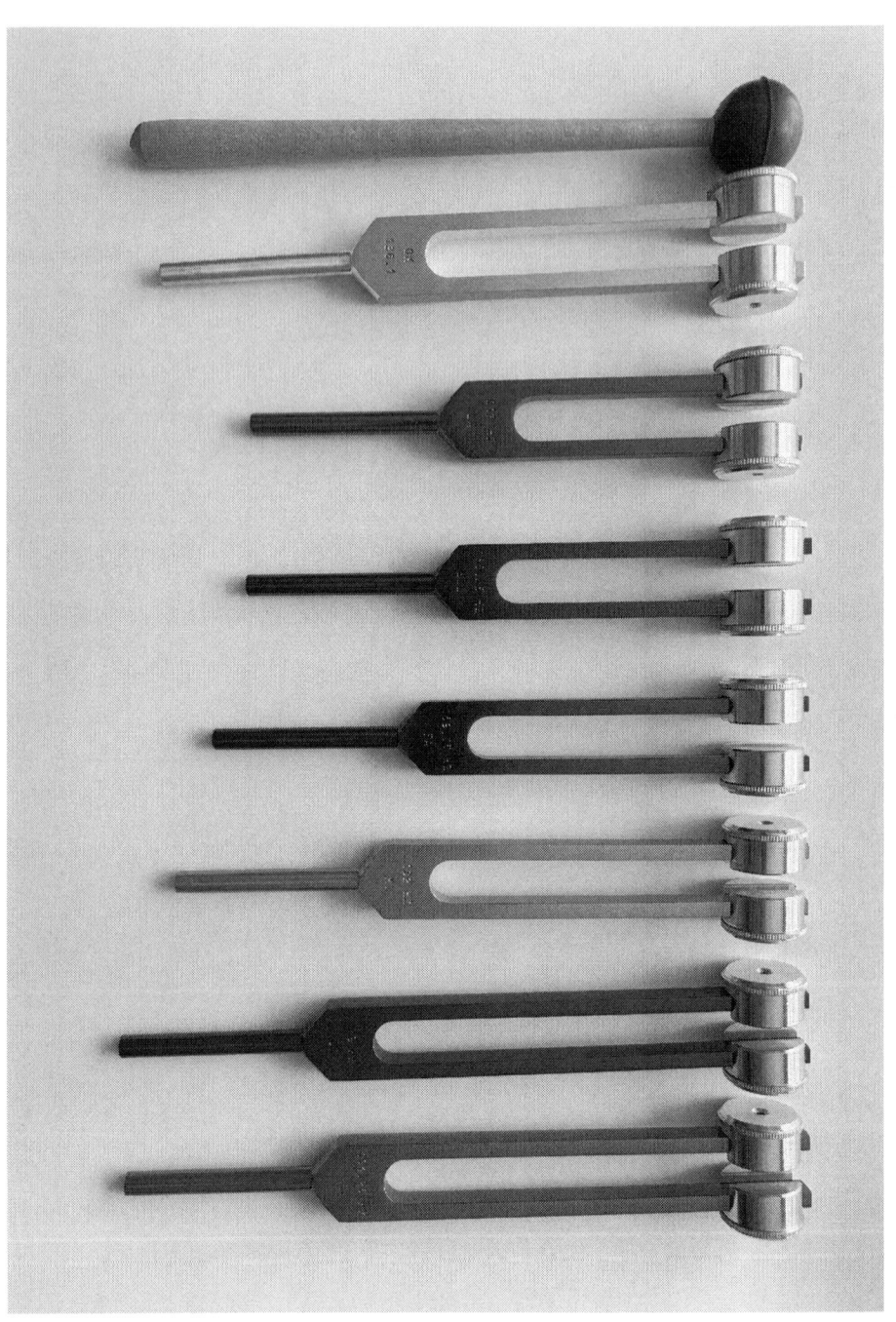

Chapter 12: Your First Tuning Fork Session

Using tuning forks for self-healing can be a powerful and effective way to promote relaxation, balance, and overall well-being.

Here are some helpful steps to select a tuning fork.

1. Choose the right tuning fork: Select a tuning fork that corresponds to the area of the body or the specific issue you want to address. For example, if you want to promote relaxation, you might choose a tuning fork that corresponds to the alpha brainwave frequency.
2. Find space that is comfortable: To get the most out of your self-healing session, it's very important to find a space that is not only comfortable but also quiet, a place where you can relax and focus on the sound of the tuning fork.
3. Strike the tuning fork: Hold the tuning fork by the stem and strike it gently against a rubber block or other hard surface. This will create a pure tone that you can use for your self-healing practice.
4. Hold the tuning fork near the body: Hold the tuning fork near the area of the body or the chakra you want to address. You can also hold the tuning fork over acupuncture points to promote energy flow.

Tuner Frequency Table

Body Tuner Frequency	Energy Tuner Frequency	Chakra	Area of Body	Energetic Imbalance
213 Hz	852 Hz	Brow (3rd Eye) Intuition	Hypothalamus, Nervous system, Brain, Head, Mouth, Eyes, Nose Pituitary Gland, Pineal Gland	Sinus problems, Blurred Vision, Nightmares, Headaches, Blindness, Eye Strain
185.25 Hz	741 Hz	Throat Communication	Throat, Larynx, Neck, Parathyroid, Thyroid, Shoulders, Esophagus	Sore throat, Neck problems, Colds, Hearing Problems, Thyroid Problems
159.75 Hz	639 Hz	Heart Connecting	Heart, Breasts, Lungs, Circulatory System, Upper arms, Respiratory System	High Blood Pressure, Asthma or other Lung Disease, Heart Disease
132 Hz	528 Hz	Solar Plexus Manifestation & Transformation	Digestive System, Adrenals, Gallbladder, Stomach, Spleen, Pancreas, Liver, Elbow	Hypoglycemia, Digestive Disorders, Gallstones, Ulcers, Diabetes
104.25 Hz	417 Hz	Sacral Change & Removal of Negative Energy	Pelvic Area, Reproductive System, Sex Glands, Bladder, Kidneys, Forearms	Uterine Problems, Kidney Problems, Bladder problems, Impotence, Fridgidity, Lower Back
99 Hz	396 Hz	Root Liberate	Base of Spine, Feet, Adrenals, Elimination System, Wrists, Hands	Sciatica, Knee Problems, Constipation, Hemorrhoids, Weight Issues, Arthritis

Listen to the sound: Close your eyes and focus on the sound of the tuning fork. Allow the sound to resonate through your body and imagine it bringing healing and balance to the area you are focusing on.

6. Repeat as needed: You can repeat the process with the same tuning fork or use different tuning forks to address different areas of the body or issues.

Remember, using tuning forks for self-healing can be a powerful tool for promoting relaxation, balance, and overall well-being. With practice and patience, you can use tuning forks to create a customized self-healing practice that works for you.

Chapter 13: Techniques

Overall, there are several different techniques that you can utilize when using tuning forks for self-healing. The key is to experiment with different techniques and find what works best for you. With practice and patience, you can create a customized self-healing practice that promotes relaxation, balance, and overall well-being. Here are some of the most popular techniques

1. Direct application: This involves holding the tuning fork directly on or near the body. For example, you might hold the tuning fork on an acupressure point or chakra to promote energy flow and balance.

2. Sound bath: This involves striking multiple tuning forks at once and allowing the sound to resonate throughout the body. This can be a powerful way to promote relaxation and balance.

3. Chakra balancing: This involves using tuning forks that correspond to each of the seven chakras to promote balance and healing in each area. You can hold the tuning fork near each chakra and focus on the corresponding sound to promote energy flow and balance.

4. Brainwave entrainment: This involves using tuning forks that correspond to different brainwave frequencies to promote relaxation, focus, or other desired states of mind. You

can hold the tuning fork near the head and focus on the corresponding sound to promote the desired state.

5. Interval training: This involves using two different tuning forks together to create an interval that promotes balance and harmony. For example, you might use a C and G tuning fork together to create a perfect fifth interval, which is believed to promote balance and harmony.

The key is to experiment with different techniques and find what works best for you. With practice and patience, you can create a customized self-healing practice that promotes relaxation, balance, and overall well-being.

Choosing the right tuning fork can be a daunting task, but it doesn't have to be! Here are some humorous tips to help you choose the perfect tuning fork for your needs:

1. Look for the right pitch: If you're looking to promote relaxation, you might want to choose a lower-pitched tuning fork. If you're looking to boost energy and focus, a higher-pitched tuning fork might be more your style. Just make sure you don't accidentally grab a fork from your kitchen drawer instead!

2. Follow your intuition: If you're not sure which tuning fork to choose, let your intuition be your guide. Close your eyes, take a deep breath, and see which tuning fork calls out to you. Just make sure you're not confusing it with the sound of your stomach growling.

3. Check the label: Tuning forks often come labeled with their corresponding frequency or chakra. If you're looking to target a specific area of the body, make sure you choose a tuning fork that matches the

corresponding frequency or chakra. And if you can't read the label, just choose the one that looks the prettiest.

4. Consider the material: Tuning forks can be made of different materials, such as aluminum, brass, or crystal. Each material can have its own unique properties and healing benefits. So, if you're feeling fancy, go for the crystal tuning fork. Just make sure you don't accidentally drop it and shatter your zen.

Chapter 14: Harmonic Frequency Tuning Forks

Harmonic frequency tuning forks are based on musical intervals and work by creating harmonious resonance within the biofield. These forks are excellent for dissolving energy blockages and establishing a coherent energy field that fosters peace and relaxation.

Key Harmonic Frequencies and Their Benefits

1. Perfect Fifth (256 Hz and 384 Hz) – A widely used harmonic pair that brings the biofield into a state of natural, alleviating anxiety and stress.
2. Perfect Fourth (512 Hz and 384 Hz) – This pair is known to bring physical and emotional relief, releasing tension and restoring a sense of calm.
3. Octave (128 Hz and 256 Hz) – This grounding pair promotes stability, making it ideal for centering oneself before or after energy work.

Step-by-Step Techniques for Using Harmonic Frequencies

Harmonizing the Biofield with the Perfect Fifth

1. Set Up a Quiet Space: Choose a comfortable, quiet place to sit or lie down.

2. Strike Both Forks Simultaneously: Hold the 256 Hz and 384 Hz tuning forks by their stems and strike them at the same time.
3. Create an Aural Field: Position one fork near each ear to allow the harmonizing sound of the Perfect Fifth to wash over you.
4. Focus on Relaxation: Close your eyes, and visualize a balanced energy field surrounding you. Feel tension dissolving with each wave of sound.
5. Deep Breathing: Inhale deeply, feeling the sound resonate within your biofield, and exhale any lingering stress.

Repeat this for five minutes or longer to enter a deeply relaxed state. This technique is highly effective in reducing stress and anxiety.

Emotional and Physical Release with the Perfect Fourth

1. Find a Relaxing Position: Sit or lie comfortably, and set an intention for emotional or physical release.
2. Strike Both Forks Together: Activate the 512 Hz and 384 Hz tuning forks simultaneously.
3. Sweep over the Body: Starting at the top of your head, slowly sweep the forks down the front and sides of your torso, paying particular attention to areas where you feel tightness or discomfort.

4. Allow the Vibration to Work: Hold the forks near any area that feels "stuck" or tense, and visualize the sound vibrations breaking up the tension.
5. Release with Breathing: Inhale deeply, then exhale, imagining the release of any tension, pain, or emotional stress.

This technique is particularly helpful for end-of-day release or after physically demanding activities.

Grounding and Centering with the Octave

1. Get Comfortable: Stand or sit with your feet firmly on the ground.
2. Activate the Octave Pair: Strike both the 128 Hz and 256 Hz tuning forks simultaneously.
3. Position at the Base of the Spine: Hold the forks on either side of the base of your spine or near your feet to promote a grounding sensation.
4. Visualize Stability: Picture yourself anchored, feeling the stability of the Earth's energy harmonizing with your own.
5. Slow Breathing: Breathe deeply and feel the connection between your body and the earth.

Use this technique as a quick grounding exercise, particularly after intense energy work or emotional release sessions.

Planetary Frequency Tuning Forks

Planetary frequency tuning forks are crafted to resonate with the vibrations of celestial bodies, each bringing a distinct energetic influence. Using these forks, we can align with the energies of the cosmos, adding depth to our spiritual and healing practices.

Key Planetary Frequencies and Their Benefits

1. Earth (136.10 Hz) – Also called the "Om" fork, this frequency resonates deeply with the Earth's natural vibration, creating grounding effects and fostering inner peace.
2. Sun (126.22 Hz) – Known for its vibrant, uplifting energy, the Sun frequency is ideal for boosting personal power, confidence, and mental clarity.
3. Moon (210.42 Hz) – This frequency supports emotional balance, intuitive awareness, and a sense of calm associated with lunar energy.

Step-by-Step Techniques for Using Planetary Frequencies

Grounding Meditation with the Earth Frequency

1. Prepare your Space: Find a quiet, comfortable spot where you won't be disturbed. Set an intention to ground and center yourself.

2. Activate the Tuning Fork: Hold the 136.10 Hz tuning fork by its stem and gently strike it with a rubber mallet.
3. Position and Hold: Bring the vibrating fork close to the base of your spine, near the root chakra. Hold it steady until the vibration fades.
4. Visualization: As you feel the vibration, visualize roots growing from your feet deep into the Earth, anchoring and stabilizing your energy.
5. Breathe Deeply: Take long, slow breaths, feeling the grounding energy of the Earth frequency absorbing into your being.

Repeat this process two to three times for a longer grounding session. The Earth frequency can also be used on the soles of the feet or near the legs to enhance a sense of rootedness.

Sun Frequency for Vitality and Confidence

1. Set the Mood: Find a well-lit space if possible, allowing sunlight to filter in to enhance the Sun frequency experience.
2. Activate the Tuning Fork: Strike the 126.22 Hz tuning fork and hold it near your solar plexus, which is the seat of personal power and energy.
3. Direct the Vibration: Place the fork about an inch from your solar plexus area. Feel the warmth and confidence radiating from the frequency.

4. Visualize Empowerment: Imagine a warm, golden light spreading from your solar plexus throughout your body, filling you with positivity, courage, and self-assurance.
5. Breathing: Breathe in deeply as you visualize, and with each exhale, release any self-doubt or lethargy.

This practice is excellent to incorporate into your morning routine or before any activity that requires confidence and vitality.

Moon Frequency for Emotional Healing and Intuition

1. Prepare the Setting: Dim the lights, light a candle, or play soft music to create a calm environment conducive to emotional release and intuition.

2. Activate the Tuning Fork: Strike the 210.42 Hz tuning fork, and hold it first at your heart chakra, then move it up to the third eye chakra.

3. Movement and Sweeping: Starting from the heart, sweep the fork in a gentle arc upward to your third eye, creating a flow of lunar energy through your emotional and intuitive centers.

4. Connect with Intuition: As the vibration moves, focus on accessing inner wisdom and compassion, allowing any emotional blocks to release.

5. Calming Breath: Take slow, calming breaths, releasing with each exhale any emotional tension or suppressed feelings.

Using the Moon frequency before sleep or during meditation enhances emotional healing and promotes intuitive insight.

Chapter 15: Choosing

Remember, choosing the right tuning fork is all about finding the one that resonates with you and your specific needs. So, don't be afraid to have a little fun and trust your instincts. And if you accidentally choose the wrong one, just use it to eat your salad instead!

Using tuning forks for self-healing can have a variety of benefits for both the mind and body. Here are some of the main benefits:

1. Reduces stress and promotes relaxation: The vibrations from the tuning forks can help to reduce stress and promote deep relaxation. This can help to calm the mind and reduce tension in the body.

2. Balances the chakras: The vibrations from the tuning forks can help to balance the energy centers in the body known as chakras. Each chakra is associated with a different aspect of the mind and body, and balancing them can promote overall well-being.

3. Promotes deep meditation: The vibrations from the tuning forks can help to deepen meditation practice and promote a more profound sense of peace and tranquility.

4. Enhances focus and concentration: Certain tuning forks can promote focus and concentration by stimulating specific brainwave frequencies.

5. Relieves pain and promotes healing: The vibrations from the tuning forks can help to relieve pain and promote healing by stimulating circulation, reducing inflammation, and promoting cellular regeneration.

6. Boosts mood and energy levels: The vibrations from the tuning forks can help to boost mood and energy levels by promoting the release of endorphins and other feel-good hormones.

Using tuning forks for self-healing can be a powerful way to promote relaxation, balance, and overall well-being. With regular practice, tuning fork therapy can help you to feel more centered, focused, and energized in both body and mind.

Chapter 16: Using Tuning Forks for Specific Ailments

Tuning forks can be an effective tool for managing pain by promoting relaxation and reducing inflammation in the body. Here are some steps for using tuning forks for pain relief:

1. Choose the right tuning fork: Select a tuning fork that is appropriate for the type of pain you are experiencing. For example, a lower frequency tuning fork may be more effective for deep, chronic pain, while a higher frequency tuning fork may be more appropriate for acute pain.

2. Identify the source of pain: Determine the area of the body where you are experiencing pain. This can help you to target the tuning fork in the correct location.

3. Strike the tuning fork: Strike the tuning fork gently on a soft surface, such as a rubber block, to create a clear, ringing sound.

4. Hold the tuning fork: Hold the base of the tuning fork against the affected area of the body, or hold it a few

inches away if the area is sensitive.

5. Feel the vibrations: Allow the vibrations from the tuning fork to permeate the affected area. You may feel a gentle tingling sensation or a warmth in the area.

6. Repeat as necessary: You can repeat the process several times, or as often as needed, to manage pain and promote relaxation

Keep in mind that tuning forks should not be used as a substitute for medical treatment. If you are experiencing severe or chronic pain, it is important to consult with a medical professional. However, tuning forks can be a helpful complementary therapy to manage pain and promote overall well being.

Chapter 17: How To Use Tuning Forks For Stress and Anxiety

1. Find space that it comfortable and quiet: Choose a space that is comfortable and quiet, a place where you won't be disturbed. This could be a quiet outdoor space or even a room in your home.
2. Select your tuning fork: Choose a tuning fork that resonates with your needs. For sleep disorders, you may want to use a fork with a lower frequency, such as an "Om" or "C" fork.
3. Strike the tuning fork against a rubber block or your knee to produce a clear, ringing sound. Make sure the fork is vibrating strongly before you move on to the next step.
4. Hold the fork: Hold the base of the fork and place the prongs against your body, starting at your forehead or the top of your head. Next, close your eyes and begin to take deep breaths.
5. Follow the vibrations: As you hold the fork against your body, follow the vibrations with your mind. Focus on the sensations and the sound of the fork. If you find that your mind begins to wander off, gently bring it back to your present moment.
6. Move the fork: Slowly move the fork down your body following the midline of your body. You can stop at any point where you feel tension or discomfort and hold the fork there for a few breaths.
7. Repeat as necessary: It is okay to repeat the process as many times as you feel that you need to, focusing on different areas of the body or using different forks

Chapter 18: Using Tuning Forks For Sleep Disorders

1. Find a space that is comfortable and quiet: Choose a quiet and comfortable space where you can lie down and relax without being disturbed.
2. Select your tuning fork: Choose a tuning fork that resonates with your needs. For sleep disorders, you may want to use a fork with a lower frequency, such as an "Om" or "C" fork.
3. Strike the fork: Strike the tuning fork against a rubber block or your knee to produce a clear, ringing sound. Make sure the fork is vibrating strongly before you move on to the next step.
4. Hold the fork: Hold the base of the fork and place the prongs against your body, starting at your forehead or the top of your head. Close your eyes and begin to take deep breaths.
5. Follow the vibrations: As you hold the fork against your body, follow the vibrations with your mind. Focus on the sensations and the sound of the fork. Imagine the sound waves traveling through your body and soothing your nervous system.
6. Move the fork: Slowly move the fork down your body, following the midline of your body. You can stop at any point where you feel tension or discomfort and hold the fork there for a few breaths.
7. Focus on your breath: Once you've finished using the tuning fork, focus on your breath and allow your body to relax completely. You may want to practice some

deep breathing exercises or progressive muscle relaxation techniques to further promote relaxation and sleep.

Chapter 19: Using Tuning Forks For Digestive Issues

1. Find a space that is comfortable and quiet: Choose a space where you can sit or lie down without being disturbed.
2. Select your tuning fork: Choose a tuning fork that resonates with your needs. For digestive issues, you may want to use a fork with a frequency that corresponds to the solar plexus chakra, such as an "E" or "A" fork.
3. Strike the fork: Strike the tuning fork against a rubber block or your knee to produce a clear, ringing sound. Make sure the fork is vibrating strongly before you move on to the next step.
4. Hold the fork: Hold the base of the fork and place the prongs against your abdomen, at or near the area where you are experiencing digestive discomfort.
5. Follow the vibrations: As you hold the fork against your abdomen, follow the vibrations with your mind. Focus on the sensations and the sound of the fork. Imagine the sound waves traveling through your digestive system and helping to promote relaxation and healing.
6. Move the fork: Slowly move the fork around your abdomen, following the path of your digestive system.

You can stop at any point where you feel tension or discomfort and hold the fork there for a few breaths.

7. This process can be repeated as many times as you like, focusing on different areas of the abdomen or using different forks

Using tuning forks for digestive issues can be a helpful way to promote relaxation and improve the functioning of your digestive system. However, it's important to remember that tuning forks should not be used as a substitute for medical treatment. If you are experiencing chronic or severe digestive issues, it's important to seek the guidance of a medical professional.

Chapter 20: How To Use Tuning Forks For Meditation and Mindfulness

1. Get into the zone: Find a quiet space, sit down and clear your mind. Maybe light a few candles or put on some soothing music to get into the mood.
2. Select your tuning fork: Choose a fork that resonates with your inner peace. Maybe one that sounds like the chimes of a fairy, or a deep and grounding tone that reminds you of your favorite barista's voice.
3. Strike the fork: Strike the tuning fork against a rubber block or a hard surface to create a pleasant and calming sound. Make sure to listen to the vibrations until they fully dissipate.
4. Close your eyes: Let the sound of the tuning fork guide you into a meditative state. Close your eyes and breathe deeply, focusing on the sound and feeling the vibrations as they wash over you.
5. Follow the sound: As the sound fades away, continue to focus on your breathing and allow your mind to become still. Use the tuning fork as a point of focus, and let it guide you towards a state of mindfulness and tranquility.
6. Repeat as necessary: Use the tuning fork whenever you need to get into the zone, or whenever you want to achieve a sense of inner peace and calm.

Using tuning forks for meditation and mindfulness can be a fun and unique way to enhance your practice. While the process may seem silly at first, the sounds and vibrations can be surprisingly effective at helping you find your center and achieve a state of mindfulness. Just remember, it's important to use the right fork for the job, so choose wisely!

Chapter 21: How To Use Tuning Forks For Chakra Balancing

1. Get in touch with your inner woo-woo: Get yourself in the right mindset by lighting some incense and putting on your comfiest pair of yoga pants.
2. Select your forks: Each chakra has its own frequency, so make sure you've got the right forks for the job. If you're not sure which fork goes where, consult your friendly neighborhood crystal healer.
3. Strike the fork: Give your fork a good tap and let it vibrate. You'll want to hear a clear and sustained tone.
4. Place the fork: Find the location of the chakra you want to balance, and place the vibrating fork on or near that area. Be careful not to poke yourself with the prongs!
5. Listen to the vibrations: Focus on the sound of the fork and feel the vibrations as they travel through your body. You can even visualize the energy flowing through the chakra as the vibrations work their magic.
6. Move on to the next chakra: Once you feel like you've spent enough time on one chakra, move on to the next one. Rinse and repeat until you feel balanced and centered.

Chapter 22: How To Use Tuning Forks For Energy Healing

1. Get in a relaxed state: Find a comfortable and quiet place where you can relax and let go of stress and tension. Sit or lie down and take some deep breaths to help you get centered and focused.

2. Choose your forks: Choose a pair of forks that have been specifically designed for energy healing. These forks typically have a higher vibration frequency and are tuned to different notes or scales to address different types of energy imbalances.

3. Activate the forks: Hold the forks by the stems and gently tap them together or against a rubber block to activate them. Once activated, place one fork on each side of the body, starting at the feet and moving upwards towards the head.

4. Listen to the sound and feel the vibrations: Listen to the sound of the forks and feel the vibrations as they travel through your body. Focus on the sensation and allow yourself to fully relax and let go of any tension or negative energy.

5. Move the forks: Slowly move the forks up and down the body, keeping them at a comfortable distance from the skin. You can also move them in a circular motion or focus on specific areas of the body that feel particularly tense or blocked.

6. Trust the process: Allow yourself to fully trust the process and believe that the forks are helping to restore balance and harmony to your energy field. Continue to listen to the sound and feel the vibrations for as long as you need to feel fully rejuvenated and energized.

Tuning forks for energy healing can be a powerful and effective way to restore balance and harmony to your energy field. By using the right forks and techniques, you can help to release tension, clear blockages, and promote a sense of overall wellbeing and vitality.

Chapter 23: Precautions To Take When Using Bio-tuning Forks

1. Avoid using tuning forks too close to the ears: While tuning forks can be used on various parts of the body, it's best to avoid using them directly on the ears as the sound vibrations can be too intense and potentially damage the ear drums.
2. Check for contraindications: Some conditions or medications may make it unsafe to use tuning forks. If you have any medical conditions or are taking any medications, consult with a healthcare provider before using tuning forks.
3. Use caution with pregnant women: Some studies suggest that high-frequency vibrations may have an impact on pregnancy, so it's best to avoid using tuning forks on or near the abdomen of pregnant women.
4. Use clean equipment: Always make sure your tuning forks are clean and free of dirt or debris before using them. If you're using them on multiple people, be sure to sterilize them in between uses.
5. Take breaks: It's important to take breaks between tuning fork sessions to allow the body to fully integrate the sound vibrations. Overusing tuning forks can lead to overstimulation and potentially cause adverse effects.

6. Listen to your body: If you experience any discomfort or pain while using tuning forks, stop immediately and consult a healthcare provider. Additionally, if you have a history of seizures or epilepsy, it's important to use tuning forks with caution.

By taking these precautions, you can ensure a safe and effective tuning fork experience. Remember to always listen to your body and seek medical advice if you have any concerns.

Here are some tips for getting the most out of your bio tuning fork practice:

1. Find a quiet and comfortable space: It's important that you find a quiet and comfortable space where you can relax and won't be disturbed. This will help you to fully relax and get the most out of your tuning fork practice.
2. Focus on your breath: Tuning fork practice can be enhanced by focusing on your breath. Take slow, deep breaths and allow yourself to fully relax and let go of any tension or stress.
3. Use intention setting: Setting an intention for your tuning fork practice can help to enhance the healing effects. Before beginning, set an intention for what you want to achieve or focus on during the practice.
4. Experiment with different techniques: There are various techniques you can use when working with tuning forks, so it's important to experiment and find what works best for you. Try different techniques, such as moving the forks in circular motions or focusing on specific areas of the body.
5. Use quality tuning forks: Using high-quality tuning forks can make a big difference in the effectiveness of your practice. Look for forks that are made with high-quality materials and have been specifically designed for bio-tuning practices.

6. Take your time: Don't rush your tuning fork practice. Take your time and allow yourself to fully relax and feel the effects of the sound vibration

7. Incorporate other practices: Tuning fork practice can be enhanced by incorporating other practices, such as meditation or yoga. Experiment with different practices and find what works best for you.

Chapter 24: How To Maintain and Care For Your Tuning Forks

Keep them clean: It's important to keep your tuning Forks clean to ensure they work properly. Give them a little soap and water bath but don't forget to towel them off so they don't catch a cold!

1. Store them properly: When you're not using your tuning forks, store them in a safe and dry place. Keep them away from any sharp objects or curious pets who might mistake them for chew toys.

2. Avoid extreme temperatures: Tuning forks can be sensitive to extreme temperatures, so it's important to avoid leaving them in hot or cold environments. They don't like to be too hot, too cold, or too lukewarm - they just want to be comfy!

3. Check for wear and tear: Over time, tuning forks can start to show signs of wear and tear. Check them regularly for any signs of damage, and if you notice anything, take them to a professional to get them fixed up.

4. Use them regularly: Tuning forks are like your favorite pair of shoes - the more you use them, the better they work. So make sure you're incorporating them into your self-care routine regularly.

5. Be gentle: Treat your tuning forks with care and respect. Don't bang them around or use excessive force when working with them. Remember, they're sensitive little creatures.

Chapter 25: Final Thoughts

In a world that can be overwhelming and chaotic at times, sound healing is a powerful tool to help us find balance and peace within ourselves. The vibrations of sound can penetrate deep into our bodies and minds, releasing tension, reducing stress, and promoting overall wellbeing.

Whether we're using tuning forks, singing bowls, or our own voices, the power of sound healing is undeniable. It can help us connect to our inner selves, open our hearts to love and compassion, and cultivate a sense of harmony and unity with the world around us.

But the true magic of sound healing lies in its ability to unlock the innate healing power within each of us. By tapping into the power of sound, we can learn to trust in our own capacity for healing and transformation, and discover a profound sense of inner peace and wellbeing.

So if you're feeling stuck, stressed, or disconnected, don't underestimate the power of sound healing to help you find your way back to a place of balance and harmony. Embrace the magic of sound, and let its gentle vibrations guide you back to a state of wholeness and wellbeing.

Dear Friend,

If you're feeling stressed, anxious, or just plain tired, it's time to take a moment for yourself. And what better way to do that than with the gentle, soothing vibrations of a bio-tuning fork?

These magical little instruments have the power to ease tension, calm the mind, and balance your energy centers. But don't take my word for it - give them a try and see for yourself!

Incorporating bio-tuning forks into your self-care routine is easy and fun. You can use them while meditating, practicing yoga, or simply relaxing on the couch. And the best part? You don't have to be a master healer to use them - anyone can benefit from their healing vibrations.

So go ahead, explore the wonderful world of bio-tuning forks. Let their gentle vibrations wash over you and soothe your soul. Your body and mind will thank you for it.

With Love, Light & Healing to You,

-- Shani R.

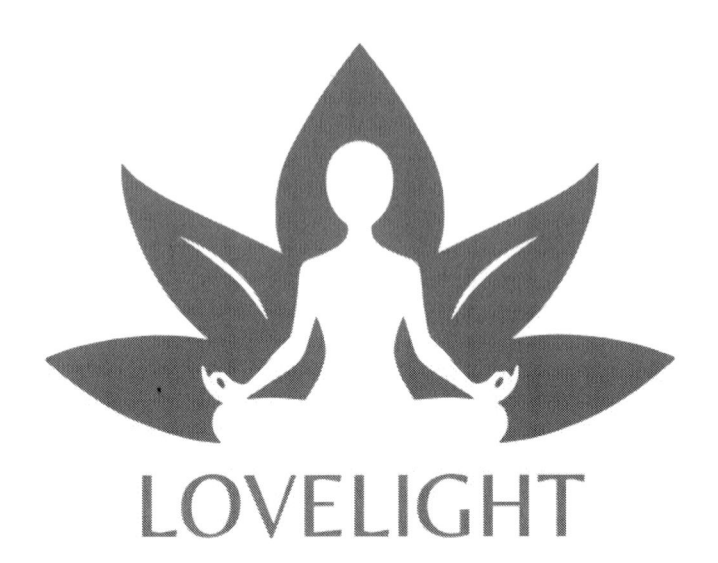

LOVELIGHT
energy healing inc
www.lovelightenergyhealinginc.com

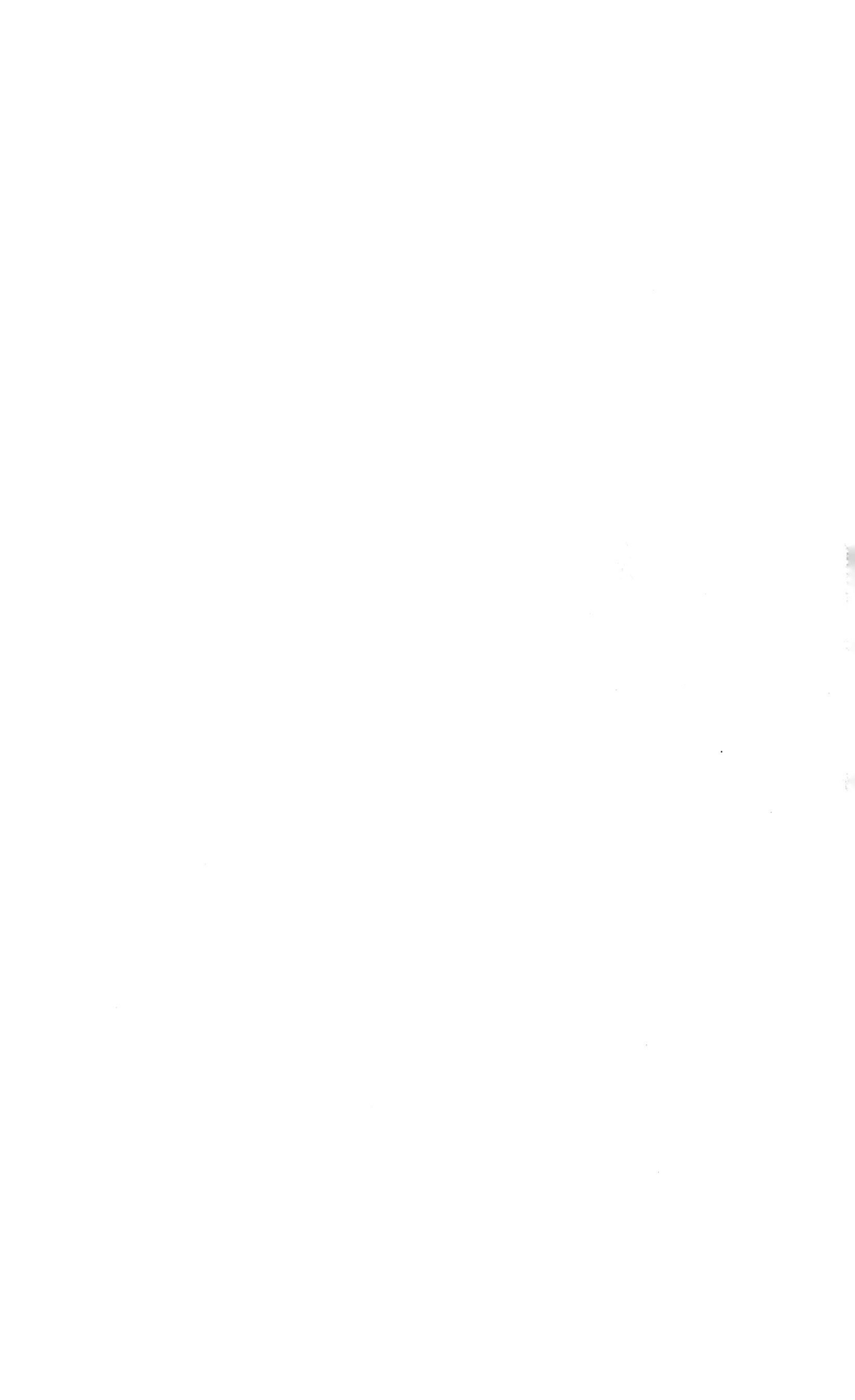

Made in United States
Troutdale, OR
09/01/2025